Perioperative care of the eye patient

Perioperative care of the eye patient

Gilli Vafidis
Consultant Ophthalmic Surgeon
the North West London Hospitals NHS Trust
Eye Unit, Central Middlesex Hospital, London

Neville Robinson
Consultant Anaesthetist
Northwick Park and St Mark's Hospitals, Middlesex

George Hall
Professor of Anaesthesia
St George's Hospital Medical School, London

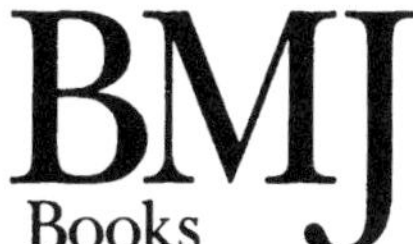

First published in 2000 by BMJ Books
BMJ Books is an imprint of the BMJ Publishing Group
BMA House, Tavistock Square, London WC1H 9JR

www.bmjbooks.com

British Library Cataloguing in Publication Data

A catalogue record for this book is available from the British Library

ISBN 0–7279–1225–9

Typeset by Phoenix Photosetting, Chatham, Kent
Printed and bound by J. W. Arrowsmith Ltd, Bristol

Contents

Preface

Success in modern ophthalmic surgery is dependent on all members of the team – nurses, surgeons and anaesthetists, understanding the important role that each individual undertakes. Unfortunately we have often found that this does not occur. The purpose of this short book is to give a brief outline of the components of care in the perioperative period that reflects current practice, with the emphasis on day stay procedures. The progression of the eye patient from surgical decisions in outpatients, to anaesthesia for the operation, to complications in the community is outlined in a way that is readily accessible to all members of the team, from consultants to operating department practitioners. It is our modest aim that each specialty will understand better the requirements of their colleagues and so enhance further the care provided for the patients.

Gilli Vafidis
Neville Robinson
George Hall

1: General preoperative assessment

All good surgery relies upon a thorough preoperative assessment. This encompasses:

- the decision to operate
- the general medical and ocular assessment
- the choice of anaesthetic, and
- relevant discussion for informed consent.

The decision to operate

In eye surgery the operation is never life saving and not often one that saves sight. The decision to operate must be taken only after the benefits of surgery have been weighed up against the risks involved.

Once surgery has been offered, the surgeon must discuss the operation, its goals and benefits with the patient. The patient should understand the advantages that the operation would confer. The elderly patient with a cataract, for example, should not be persuaded to have cataract surgery if there is no identified need. If, however, better eyesight is needed, the likely outcome and possible complications of surgery must be discussed in non-medical language before a final decision is made.

General benefits of eye surgery

The indications for eye surgery are shown in Box 1.1.

Box 1.1 Indications for eye surgery

- To improve the quality of vision
- To improve the ocular symptoms of an individual
- To prevent further deterioration of eye function
- To improve the appearance of an individual

Most eye operations are performed to improve the quality of vision by clearing opacities from the visual axis (cornea, lens or vitreous). Cataract surgery is the commonest operation in this category and is currently one of the most effective of all surgical interventions. Other frequently performed operations are those that, while conferring no immediate visual benefit, prevent deterioration of vision in the long term. Some elderly patients may not consider surgery justifiable for long-term goals.

The choice of anaesthetic

The decision about the type of anaesthesia (local or general) is often discussed when the decision to proceed with the operation is made, and this choice will influence the preoperative assessment. The preferences of both patient and ophthalmologist are important. Although local anaesthesia is possible for nearly all eye surgery, it is imperative that the patient understands its implications. Conversion to general anaesthesia, or the use of sedation during surgery, may adversely affect the outcome and is to be avoided whenever possible. For local anaesthesia, the patient needs to be reassured that there will be total analgesia during surgery and that the operation will not be hindered by being awake.

General risks of eye surgery

There are risks inherent in all surgical procedures and anaesthetic techniques. Although they may be increased by coexisting pathology, they can be minimised by good preparation of the patient. Ocular and systemic factors need to be considered so that problems are minimised during and after eye surgery (Box 1.2).

In general, surgery should be postponed if the patient's general medical condition can be improved. Some patients have poor general health, but are on optimal treatment for their illness and are unlikely to be improved if surgery is delayed. Risk versus benefit assessment in these cases needs to be carried out carefully.

Aims of the preoperative assessment

Conditions need to be optimal for the proposed operation. There are three possible problem areas: eye problems, general health problems, and social factors. An appropriate history and examination, when combined with relevant investigations, must be made to assess perioperative risks. The guidelines are summarised in Box 1.3.

Box 1.2 Factors that increase risks in eye surgery

- Eye
  - active infection in eye or elsewhere – skin ulcers, gum abscess
  - uncontrolled hypertension – risk of expulsive haemorrhage in intraocular surgery
  - anticoagulation – risk of excessive bleeding
  - uncontrolled violent behaviour – risk of postoperative wound rupture
- General medical
  - uncontrolled/poorly controlled systemic disease
  - recent myocardial infarction – within 3 months of uncomplicated myocardial infarction
  - uncontrolled blood glucose (> 12 mmol/litre) in previously undiagnosed/poorly treated diabetes
  - recent cerebrovascular accident – within 3 months

Box 1.3 Guidelines for preoperative assessment

- If the problems are temporary, for example conjunctivitis or upper respiratory tract infection, surgery is postponed.
- If there is a chronic illness, eye surgery is undertaken when the condition is stable on optimal treatment.
- If general anaesthesia is indicated, there should be a full anaesthetic assessment by the anaesthetist.
- Poor social circumstances need to be identified so that admission can be planned with increased home support in the immediate postoperative period.

Patient information

This is an important component of the preoperative assessment. Written information is used to supplement and reinforce the consultation. The visually impaired need alternative sources of information, and tape recorded or video information can be useful. Examples of preoperative patient information leaflets are given in Appendices A and B.

Informed consent

Written consent is a legal requirement for all surgical procedures (see Box 1.4). Informed consent means that the patient has adequate information and understanding about the surgery before signing the consent form. It is mandatory for the surgeon to discuss the proposed operation, its anticipated outcome and risks, and the major hazards of anaesthesia. The detail required will depend on the patient's understanding and curiosity. A well-informed and forewarned patient has more realistic surgical expectations and a better outcome. In addition, obtaining informed consent is an important component of risk management, and may prevent the pursuit of medical negligence claims if things go wrong.

Box 1.4 Essential components of consent

- Name of the patient
- Name of the doctor
- Name of the procedure, clearly legible
- If unilateral surgery planned, the eye/side must be indicated
- Signature of the patient
- Signature of the doctor
- Date

2: Specific assessment and investigation

The specific assessment depends on the planned operation, the chosen anaesthetic and the medical conditions that coexist. This chapter discusses some of the problems that often arise in eye surgery (Box 2.1).

Box 2.1 Preoperative assessment of the eye: key features

- Known antibiotic allergy will alter the postoperative antibiotic regimen.
- Active infection or inflammation must be controlled before surgery.
- The surgeon must know about previous eye or lid surgery and any coexisting eye conditions.

Cataract surgery

This is the commonest eye operation. In addition to assessment features listed in Box 2.1, the following findings will alter the preoperative or operative management.

- Poor corneal endothelial function will need added protection during surgery.
- Poor pupil dilation will require iris hooks or sphincterotomy.
- Active diabetic retinopathy reduces successful outcome and must be treated before surgery.
- In large eye (high myopia) or known scleral bulge, avoid retrobulbar injection of local anaesthetic.
- Retained fluid in lacrimal sac (mucocoele) requires antibiotics and possible sac excision before surgery.

Investigation for cataract surgery

Specific investigation includes biometry measurements for intraocular lens power. Unexpected or oblique keratometry readings may indicate corneal pathology, or influence incision placement. Ultrasound globe readings showing length > 25 mm or < 20 mm must be checked in order to avoid errors in intraocular lens calculation.

Systemic assessment and investigation

Often eye surgery is conducted on patients who are at the extremes of age. The elderly may have medical diseases that present at assessment either as undiagnosed, inadequately treated, or untreated. If left inadequately managed, these conditions cause increased patient morbidity and can adversely affect the outcome of surgery.

Diabetes mellitus

This syndrome, characterised by hyperglycaemia, is typically classified as Type 1 (insulin-dependent diabetes mellitus, IDDM) or Type 2 (non-insulin-dependent diabetes mellitus, NIDDM). The complications of diabetes are shown in Box 2.2.

There is strong evidence that good glycaemic control delays the onset and decreases the severity of microvascular complications. Unfortunately it does not influence the macrovascular complications. The adequacy of control of diabetes can be assessed, if necessary, by measuring the circulating glycosylated haemoglobin (HbA_1C) concentration. Surgery and anaesthesia can cause serious problems with glucose homeostasis in poorly controlled diabetics.

Box 2.2 Complications of diabetes mellitus

- Macrovascular
    cerebrovascular disease
    coronary artery disease
    peripheral vascular disease
- Microvascular
    nephropathy
    neuropathy – somatic, autonomic
    retinopathy – background, maculopathy, preproliferative, proliferative, advanced
- Skin
- Increased risk of infection

Refer these patients back to their general practitioner or to the local hospital diabetic clinic for improved control before proceeding with surgery. In undiagnosed patients a random urine sample which shows glycosuria is suggestive, but not diagnostic, of diabetes. A fasting blood glucose concentration >6.1 mmol/litre (7.0 mmol/litre on a plasma sample) confirms the diagnosis. The surgery should be postponed and the patient referred to the appropriate diabetic clinic for further management.

The anaesthetic management of well-controlled diabetic patients (HbA$_1$C <10%) is outlined in Box 2.3. Since both hypoglycaemia and hyperglycaemia must be avoided and are clinically undetectable under general anaesthesia, we recommend regional anaesthesia whenever possible. Many regimens exist and the following is easy to apply.

Box 2.3 Anaesthetic management of diabetic patients

- Regional anaesthesia preferable
- Ideally, first case on morning list
- Monitor blood glucose before, during, and after operation (may need to be hourly)
- Diet controlled: as normal patient
- Tablet controlled: continue medication on day (**NB** Some drugs have long half-lives and delayed hypoglycaemia can occur –chlorpropamide should be omitted)
- Insulin:
  morning list – no morning insulin, usual insulin and food after surgery
  afternoon list – usual morning insulin and light breakfast on day of surgery with usual food and insulin after surgery
- Consider "sliding scale" if poor control:
  intravenous 5% or 10% glucose infusion, 1 litre/12 h with intravenous soluble insulin 1–4 units/h depending on hourly blood glucose values

---

Cardiovascular disease

Patients with well-controlled ischaemic disease should take all their cardiac drugs on the day of operation. **This is an important principle that must be adhered to.**

Patients may come for assessment with known cardiac disease, but it is not uncommon for undiagnosed problems to present at this time. Elderly patients often have occasional ectopic beats and these are usually benign in nature. Many patients have conduction defects. Atrial fibrillation often presents as an incidental finding and occurs in about 5% of people over 65 years of age. About half will have associated ischaemic heart disease, mitral stenosis, hypertension or cardiomyopathy but often no cause is found. Atrial fibrillation is potentially hazardous. A fast rate decreases cardiac output and this arrhythmia makes patients prone to emboli. Such patients should be treated (normally with an antiarrhythmic such as amiodarone, and often by anticoagulation) before surgery. First degree heart block usually needs no further investigation. Patients with second and third degree heart block should be referred to a cardiologist before surgery and many of these patients will need cardiac pacing.

Patients with valvular disease often have a fixed cardiac output that is incapable of responding to the haemodynamic changes associated with general anaesthesia; this is especially so with aortic and mitral stenosis. These patients may also be on anticoagulant therapy.

Anticoagulation

Stopping anticoagulant therapy before surgery increases the risk of the patient having a thromboembolic complication (transient ischaemic attack, cerebrovascular accident, or pulmonary embolism). The risk must be balanced against the risk of eye haemorrhage if anticoagulation is not stopped. Since the risk of haemorrhage in eye surgery is low, it is now recommended that anticoagulation treatment is continued throughout the operative period, for as long as the prothrombin time is less than twice normal (international normalised ratio (INR) <2).

Patients with a history of cerebrovascular disease often take drugs such as aspirin. Although aspirin has been associated with extensive periorbital bleeding in eyelid surgery, the benefit probably outweighs the risk of intraocular haemorrhage in intraocular surgery and it is usually continued throughout the operative period. An individual risk analysis is indicated if lid surgery is contemplated.

Hypertension

Hypertension can be defined from the therapeutic point of view as a blood pressure > 160/90 mmHg when the patient is seated; the recordings are made on several different occasions in a quiet room with well-maintained, calibrated equipment with a cuff of appropriate size. The diastolic pressure is that recorded when there is disappearance of audible sounds (phase V). The aim of treatment should be a blood pressure < 160/90 in all patients under 80 years of age. The consequences of inadequate treatment include cerebrovascular accident, myocardial infarction, renal and cardiac failure, and retinopathy. General anaesthesia in hypertensive patients can cause major swings in blood pressure and hypertension should be well controlled before surgery is considered.

Furthermore, very high blood pressure is associated with an increased risk of choroidal haemorrhage (expulsive haemorrhage) during intraocular surgery, even under local anaesthesia. Surgery must be postponed in inadequately treated hypertensive patients.

Patients often have high initial blood pressure values at the preoperative assessment clinic and repeated measurements should be made to verify any abnormalities.

Cerebral disease

Some elderly patients have dementia, mild or severe, which can cause confusion. However, a confused patient may have any one of a number of medical problems, some of which are treatable (Box 2.4).

Lung disease

Patients undergoing surgery with regional anaesthesia must be

---

Box 2.4 Common causes of confusion in the elderly

- Hypoxia and hypercarbia – cardiac failure
- Infection – pneumonia
- Metabolic – uraemia, electrolyte disturbances, thyroid disease
- Central nervous system disorders – degeneration
- Sensory deprivation – visual, auditory impairment
- Sensory overload – pain, constipation, urinary retention
- Temperature abnormalities – hypothermia
- Drugs - alcohol, and especially cardiovascular and central nervous system drugs.

---

able to lie flat and still without coughing. Those with chronic bronchitis and asthma need to be free of infection and may require intensive physiotherapy preoperatively. General anaesthesia may be contraindicated in patients with emphysema because of the risk of pneumothorax from rupture of a lung bulla.

Diseases of relevance to anaesthesia

Even when surgery is contemplated under regional anaesthesia, it is possible that sedation or general anaesthesia will be needed. It is important to inform the anaesthetist of all relevant findings on the preoperative assessment. A history of plasma cholinesterase deficiency, drug allergies, inherited muscle disorders, and family history of malignant hyperthermia, have special relevance to anaesthesia. We recommend that the anaesthetist is informed about all patients with serious medical problems undergoing eye surgery, even if anaesthesia is performed by the eye surgeon.

Investigation

Investigations are performed to screen for unrecognised disease and to further investigate known disease. A careful history and clinical examination will indicate the appropriate investigation(s). A basic guide is shown in Box 2.5.

Box 2.5 Investigations before surgery

- All patients: heart rate, blood pressure, temperature and urinalysis
- All premenopausal patients undergoing general anaesthesia: haemoglobin
- African-Caribbean patients: haemoglobin electrophoresis for sickle cell disease
- Electrocardiogram: patients >60 years and those with cardiac history
- Chest x-ray: patients >60 years, smokers, recent immigrants
- Plasma electrolytes: if relevant clinical and drug history

3: Surgical decisions

There are four indications for surgery to the eye and orbit:

- to improve vision
- to reduce symptoms
- to prevent loss of vision, and
- to enhance appearance.

To avoid unnecessary complications, both the patient and the eye(s) need to be in optimal condition for surgery.

Elective or emergency

Eye operations are rarely emergencies. The degree of urgency depends on whether the patient's vision will be made worse if surgery is delayed. This occurs in a few instances, such as penetrating eye injuries and retinal detachment, when immediate surgery must be considered. Emergency eye surgery should not be undertaken if it poses an unacceptable risk to the patient's life, and must be deferred until the patient's medical problem(s) can be stabilised (Box 3.1).

Box 3.1 Factors that may delay emergency or elective surgery

- Anaesthetic – full stomach, previous anaesthetic complications
- Surgical – trauma involving other systems
- Acute medical conditions – acute heart failure, asthma
- Chronic medical disease – uncontrolled/untreated disease such as diabetes mellitus
- Eye and orbit problems
    inflammation
    infection

Day stay or overnight stay

Inpatient surgery is becoming less common, but there are still some indications for this type of surgery (Box 3.2).

Uncomplicated eye surgery needs neither observation nor intervention by the ophthalmic team. Unexpected complications, however, may require inpatient care in the immediate postoperative period. Following general anaesthesia, systemic conditions may need inpatient monitoring that could have been avoided if regional anaesthesia had been used. It is important to foresee this eventuality.

Box 3.2 Indications for inpatient surgery

- Ophthalmic – perioperative monitoring and treatment
- Anaesthetic – general anaesthetic assessment and complications
- Medical conditions – such as homozygous sickle cell anaemia
- Social factors

The most common indication for inpatient care is social. There are no hard and fast rules about who should undergo ambulatory regional anaesthesia, but it is considered preferable for patients to have someone at home on the first postoperative night and to have independent transport to and from the day-care unit. In the elderly, poor home support and dependence on public transport may rule out day care unless innovative solutions are considered with adequate preplanning of admission and discharge arrangements (Box 3.3).

Box 3.3 Social factors and their solutions

- No transport
    provide transport to and from day centre
    postoperative review at site close to patient
- No home support
    portable telephone for communication with hospital
    home visit by ophthalmic/practice nurse on first postoperative day
    low dependency, or hotel accommodation, provided overnight

---

Regional or general anaesthesia

Most routine eye operations can be undertaken with regional anaesthesia. Pain is controlled adequately, and surgical access is excellent with the patient's co-operation. The absolute and relative contraindications to regional anaesthesia are shown in Box 3.4.

Box 3.4 Contraindications to regional anaesthesia

- Patient's refusal
- Children up to the age of "early teens"
- Psychiatric and psychological problems:
    mental retardation
    claustrophobia
    senile dementia
    needle phobia
- Head movements or tremors – Parkinson's disease
- Communication difficulties – deafness, language
- Inability to lie flat
- Surgery >2 hours' duration
- Emergency surgery – penetrating eye injury
- Surgeon's preference for general anaesthesia
- Allergy to local anaesthetic drugs

Regional anaesthesia offers many advantages over general anaesthesia (Box 3.5) and, in practice, is contraindicated in very few patients. Most should be encouraged to have eye surgery with this technique, although a few will need reassurance that the

---

Box 3.5 Advantages of regional anaesthesia

- Faster recovery
- Avoids the complications of general anaesthesia
- Less nausea and vomiting
- Early discharge from hospital
- Better postoperative analgesia
- Blocks the oculocardiac reflex
- Usual mental status retained
- Patient retains "control"
- Less expensive

---

surgeon and theatre team are happy with local anaesthesia. Some patients benefit from discussing the experience with other patients who have had eye surgery under regional anaesthesia.

General anaesthesia has a few advantages over regional anaesthesia (Box 3.6).

Box 3.6 Advantages of general anaesthesia

- Preferable with some psychological, medical, and surgical conditions
- Suitable for all ages
- Avoids complications of regional anaesthesia
    retrobulbar haemorrhage
    globe perforation
    myotoxicity
    brainstem anaesthesia
    failed block
- May be preferable for teaching surgical techniques

A checklist for surgical decisions can be found in Appendix C.

Starvation before surgery

When general anaesthesia is used, patients must have an empty stomach. They should be starved for 4–6 hours preoperatively. Unfortunately this does not guarantee that the stomach is empty. For emergency surgery, especially after trauma, gastric emptying is delayed and patients have been known to vomit a complete meal 12 hours later.

Guidance for regional anaesthesia is more controversial and some units have policies allowing unrestricted food and fluid ingestion before surgery – this may be beneficial in patients with diabetes – but the management of the major complications of regional anaesthesia, and indeed the conversion of an operation under local anaesthesia to general anaesthesia, is fraught with the risk of aspiration of gastric contents. Therefore, a safe policy for regional anaesthesia is to use the same guidelines for preoperative starvation as for general anaesthesia.

4: Regional anaesthesia

Successful regional anaesthesia implies adequate analgesia and immobility of the globe and eyelids (akinesia) to create conditions for safe surgery. Several techniques are used and this chapter outlines the most common, their indications and side effects, and discusses what to do when they fail.

Anatomy

Figure 4.1 shows the anatomy of the eye and orbit. The perfect ocular local anaesthetic would block four motor (III, IV, VI,VII),

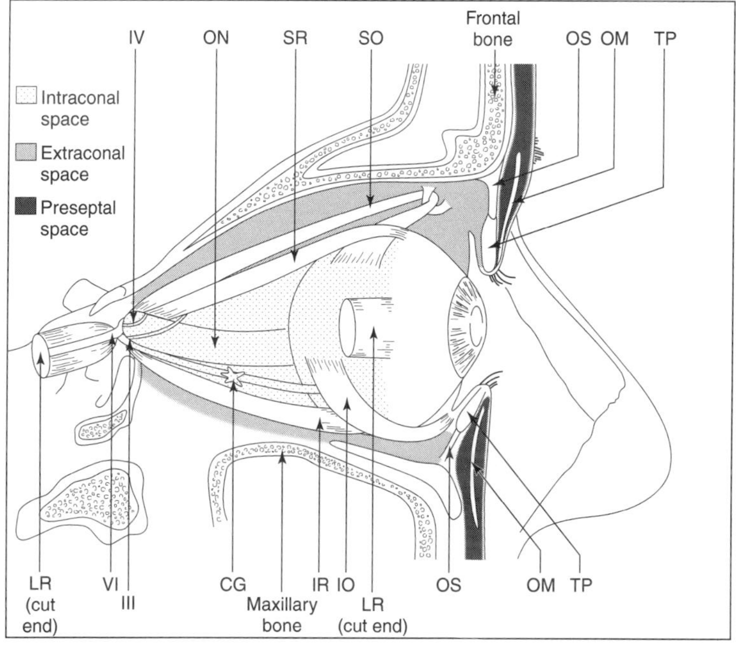

Figure 4.1 Anatomy of the eye and orbit.
Abbreviations. Nerves: III 3rd cranial nerve (superior and inferior divisions); IV 4th cranial nerve; VI 6th cranial nerve; ON optic nerve (2nd cranial nerve); CG ciliary ganglion (parasympathetic). Muscles: LR lateral rectus; IR inferior rectus; SR superior rectus; IO inferior oblique; SO superior oblique; OM orbicularis muscle; OS orbital septum. Eyelid: TP tarsal plate.

and three sensory (II, V1,V2) cranial nerves, as well as the autonomic nerve supply to the orbit. Since most ophthalmic nerves pass through the apex of the orbit, the anaesthetic must reach the posterior orbit if it is to achieve complete analgesia and akinesia. A total nerve block is not always necessary and the anaesthetic can be modified to suit the operation by the targeting of specific orbital spaces for the local analgesic.

The anterior and posterior orbit is divided into preseptal and postseptal spaces by a vertically aligned septum. The postseptal space contains the rectus muscles which form the boundary of the retrobulbar space (the intraconal space). Since the retrobulbar space contains the autonomic ciliary ganglion, the ophthalmic veins and many relevant nerves, including the optic nerve, injection into this space produces rapid, effective anaesthesia.

Outside the rectus cone, in the postseptal space, is the extra-conal compartment into which a peribulbar injection is given. This space contains few nerves, and peribulbar anaesthesia works by diffusion into the retrobulbar space. A larger volume of anaesthetic is needed, up to 10 ml.

Preseptal anaesthesia affects pain sensation from periorbital skin and some conjunctiva but does not reach the nerves serving eye movements, vision, pupillary reactions, and deep pain. Therefore it is often inadequate for major eye surgery.

Operative preparation

Correct assessment and patient preparation is fundamental for successful regional anaesthesia. Informed consent for both surgery and anaesthesia must be obtained. Surgery should only take place after an indwelling intravenous cannula has been inserted and where there is access to full monitoring and resuscitation equipment.

Which regional anaesthetic technique?

Simple is best. A compromise is necessary between using the least invasive technique, that has minimal complications, and satisfactory anaesthesia. Currently there are four principal approaches to ocular anaesthesia and these are classified according to the site of application of the local anaesthetic. The risk to major orbital structures and of life-threatening complications increases through techniques 1 to 4:

1. *Surface (topical) anaesthesia*: affects conjunctiva and cornea (skin), and is indicated for foreign body removal, superficial biopsy, ocular injections, and some cataract surgery.

2. *Subcutaneous (subconjunctival) anaesthesia*: affects skin and anterior globe, causing akinesia of lids and periorbital muscles, and is indicated for lid surgery and some muscle, cataract, and lacrimal surgery.

3. *Peribulbar anaesthesia*: affects the globe causing akinesia of the globe and pupil, and is indicated for cataract, glaucoma, and some vitreoretinal surgery.

4. *Retrobulbar anaesthesia*: affects the globe causing akinesia of the globe and pupil, and is indicated for cataract, glaucoma and some vitreoretinal surgery.

These regional techniques can be modified so that the efficacy of the block is maintained whilst the risk and discomfort to the patient are decreased. The regional anaesthetic techniques used by the authors are outlined below.

Topical (surface) anaesthesia

Local anaesthetic (e.g. amethocaine 0.5%, proxymetacaine 0.5%) drops are placed on the cornea, conjunctiva, or lid margin. The block may be modified by the use of local anaesthetic (2% lignocaine)-soaked sponges placed in the inferior or superior fold of the conjunctiva to provide more sustained analgesia. The characteristics of this technique are shown in Box 4.1.

Subcutaneous or subconjunctival anaesthesia

A 27G sharp needle is inserted under the skin or conjunctiva and 1–7 ml of local anaesthetic (2% lignocaine) are slowly

---

Box 4.1 Characteristics of topical anaesthesia

- Nerves affected – sensory: superficial branches of V1 and V2
- Advantages – safe, easy to perform, rapid onset
- Disadvantages – only superficial analgesia, no akinesia
- Supplemental use – commonly used with other regional techniques
- Recovery time – < 1 h, depending on the local anaesthetic used
- Complications – rarely corneal epithelial damage (multiple drops in unhealthy cornea)

infiltrated to raise a small bleb. The bleb can be massaged to reduce swelling in the eye and aid diffusion of the local anaesthetic. Modifications include warming the local anaesthetic to try to reduce the pain of the injection. Adrenaline 1:200 000 can be added to the local anaesthetic to prolong the block and to reduce bleeding. The characteristics of this block are shown in Box 4.2.

Box 4.2 Characteristics of subconjunctival or subcutaneous anaesthesia

- Nerves affected

    Subconjunctival – sensory: pain fibres to skin and eye of V1 and V2

    Subcutaneous – sensory: VI and V2; motor: periocular fibres VII
- Advantages – good analgesia for lid surgery and superficial ocular procedures where topical anaesthesia is insufficient
- Disadvantages – painful and can cause periorbital bruising
- Supplemental use – in cataract surgery can reduce the "squeezing" effect of orbicularis muscle around lids
- Recovery time – normal sensation <3 h, bruising about 1 week
- Complications – rarely damage to superficial tissues, globe perforation

---

Peribulbar anaesthesia

This is the most frequently used local anaesthetic block because of its simplicity and efficacy; it is an injection into the extraconal space. The injection is given with the patient lying flat and the gaze in the primary position (optic nerve on the nasal side of the mid-sagittal plane of the visual axis) (Figure 4.2).

A 27G flexible needle is passed through the skin at the junction of the middle and outer third of the inferior orbital rim. The needle is directed at right angles to the coronal plane with the tip angled at 30 degrees medially. The needle is inserted 1 cm and then gently curved upwards, avoiding the orbital floor and angled towards the middle of the head. The needle is further inserted 1–2 cm and then aspirated. If no blood is encountered, 5–7 ml of plain bupivacaine 0.5% is slowly injected. The patient experiences a mild stinging and pressure sensation as the injection is given. A swelling in the medial upper orbit may become apparent with lowering of the upper eyelid as the anaesthetic becomes effective. After the needle has been

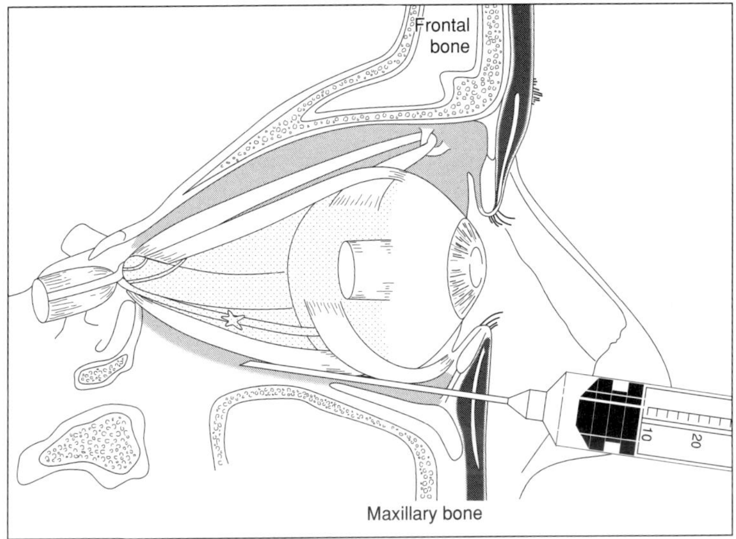

Figure 4.2 Peribulbar injection

withdrawn, orbital pressure should be administered for a few minutes before the start of surgery to reduce intraorbital pressure.

The block can be modified by injecting through the inferior conjunctiva rather than skin. Adrenaline (1:200 000) and hyaluronidase (7.5 units/ml) may be added to increase the efficacy and duration of the block. The injection can be warmed and diluted to reduce discomfort to the patient. Further injections are sometimes given to the superior and medial extraconal space in an attempt to improve the quality of the block. The characteristics of this block are described in Box 4.3.

Box 4.3 Characteristics of peribulbar anaesthesia

- Nerves affected – sensory: II, V1,V2; motor: III, IV, VI, partial VII, parasympathetic, sympathetic
- Advantages – less risk of globe perforation than retrobulbar block, no risk of optic nerve perforation if needle inserted < 3 cm
- Disadvantages – swelling around the eye may hinder surgery, risk of myotoxicity from large volume of local anaesthetic
- Recovery time – about 6 h
- Complications – globe perforation, retrobulbar haemorrhage

Retrobulbar anaesthesia

Retrobulbar injection is no longer as widely used as peribulbar and subtenons anaesthesia (see below) because of its association with an increased risk of globe perforation. The characteristics of this block are shown in Box 4.4.

Box 4.4 Characteristics of retrobulbar anaesthesia

- Nerves affected – sensory: II,V1,V2; motor: III, IV, VI, and partial VII, parasympathetic, sympathetic
- Advantages – excellent anaesthesia
- Disadvantages – a skilled technique supplemented by a facial nerve block that leaves the patient with a temporary weakness of the ipsilateral side of the face
- Contraindications – large eyes, myopic bulges (staphylomas) increase the risk of globe perforation if a sharp needle is used
- Recovery time – <6 h
- Complications – globe perforation, retrobulbar haemorrhage

The technique is described with the patient lying flat with the gaze in the primary position (Figure 4.3). A 27G needle is passed through the skin at the junction of the middle and outer third of the inferior orbital rim. The shaft of the needle is directed superomedially towards the middle of head. At 3 cm depth, the needle is aspirated and, if there is no blood, 3–5 ml 0.5% bupivacaine is slowly injected. The needle is withdrawn and the globe massaged to reduce intraocular pressure.

A facial nerve block (subcutaneous injection lateral to orbit, or infiltration of facial nerve at the angle of jaw) is given to prevent muscle contraction around the eye during surgery which increases orbital pressure.

The block can be modified by the use of a flat bevelled needle to reduce the risk of ocular perforation. Adrenaline (1:200 000) and hyaluronidase (7.5 units/ml) may be added to the injection to increase the efficacy of the block. The solution may be warmed and diluted to reduce patient discomfort.

The **subtenons technique** is an alternative to retrobulbar injection and avoids the use of a sharp cannula and therefore the risk of globe perforation. A passage is cut through the conjunctiva

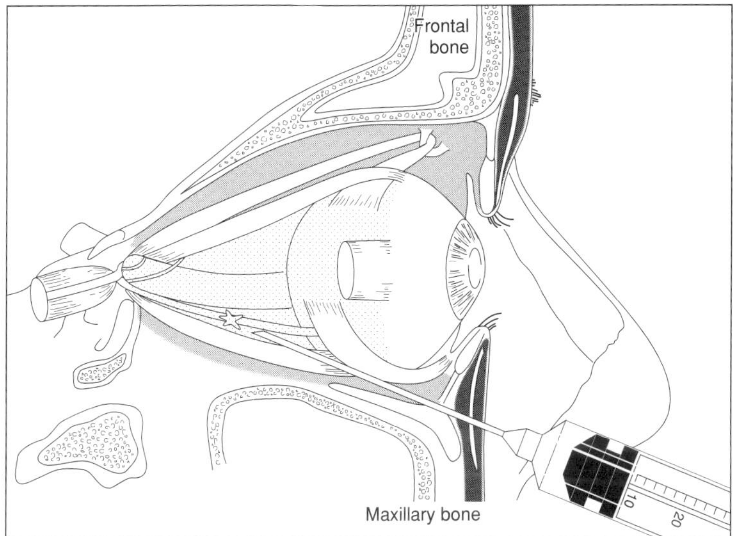

Figure 4.3 Retrobulbar injection

and subconjunctival tissue between the medial and inferior rectus muscles before local anaesthesia is injected into the retrobulbar space with a blunt cannula. This technique is gaining popularity. It requires experience of handling conjunctiva but has the great advantage of avoiding the risk of globe perforation.

Complications of regional anaesthesia

The mechanisms of the major complications of anaesthetic injection into the orbit are shown in Box 4.5.

Sedation

No regional anaesthetic technique can be guaranteed to produce ideal surgical conditions. For some surgeons this is a potent argument for using sedation. In our experience sedation is unnecessary if the patient is adequately assessed and counselled before surgery.

Box 4.5 Complications of anaesthetic injections into the orbit

- Orbital vein puncture or tearing leading to haemorrhage and retrobulbar haematoma
- Orbital artery puncture or tearing leading to massive haemorrhage, retrobulbar haematoma, and ischaemia
- Occlusion of the central retinal artery from retrobulbar or intrasheath haematoma
- Optic nerve penetration directly from local anaesthetic spread, or ischaemic compression, or trauma, leading to transient or permanent visual field loss and possible optic atrophy
- Globe penetration or perforation from needle insertion leading to pain, globe hypotony during surgery, intraocular haemorrhage, and possible retinal detachment
- Optic nerve sheath penetration with injection of local anaesthetic leading to brainstem anaesthesia – apnoea, hypotension
- Accidental intravenous and intra-arterial injection leading to convulsions, possible asystole
- Needle insertion may elicit the oculocardiac reflex with bradycardia and hypotension
- Extraocular muscle palsies from direct injection into the muscles themselves
- Facial nerve palsy

Management of failure of regional anaesthesia

If regional anaesthesia fails before surgery starts, the operation should be postponed and rebooked, for either a second regional anaesthetic or for general anaesthesia.

Unfortunately regional anaesthesia is not universally acceptable to every patient once surgery has started. There are three options to manage this problem. Firstly, if the patient is experiencing pain, a top-up of local anaesthetic may be beneficial. Topical anaesthetic or a subconjunctival injection of 2–4 ml of lignocaine 2% can help. Secondly, if the patient is anxious and cannot co-operate with surgery, sedation with 1–2 mg increments of intravenous midazolam can be given. Thirdly, general anaesthesia may be a last resort.

5: General anaesthesia

Patients requiring general anaesthesia need a full medical history and examination. This usually involves all members of the interdisciplinary team: nurses, ophthalmologists, and anaesthetists. The definition of fitness for general anaesthesia is difficult: it depends upon the urgency of the situation. For example, a patient who has life-threatening injuries is deemed fit for anaesthesia irrespective of any pre-existing medical conditions (Box 5.1).

Box 5.1 Classification of operations

- Emergency: immediate life-saving operation within one hour of surgical consultation
- Urgent: operation as soon as possible after resuscitation, usually within 24 hours of surgical consultation
- Scheduled: early operation between 1 and 3 weeks, which is not immediately life-saving
- Elective: operation at a time to suit both the patient and the surgeon

---

Most eye operations are scheduled or elective but can be urgent and occasionally are emergency procedures. They are often considered urgent when sight is threatened. It is sometimes difficult to convey an overall impression of the complexity of a patient's medical condition and anaesthetists often refer to one of the five American Society of Anesthesiologists' (ASA) Physical Status Classes (Box 5.2). This classification does not consider factors such as age, and the nature and duration of any intended surgery.

It is very unusual for a patient with an ASA grading of 4 or more to be considered for eye surgery.

Preoperative assessment for general anaesthesia

History

Age, present illness, drugs, allergies, past anaesthetic and operative history, anaesthetic family history, and social (smoking,

Box 5.2 ASA Physical Status Classes

- ASA1: normal healthy patient
- ASA2: patient with mild controlled systemic disease that does not affect normal activity, such as mild hypertension and mild diabetes
- ASA3: patient with severe systemic disease that limits activity, such as angina and chronic bronchitis
- ASA4: patient with incapacitating systemic disease that is a constant threat to life
- ASA5: moribund patient who is not expected to survive 24 hours either with, or without, an operation
- E: emergency procedure

alcohol) aspects constitute patient history. For example, current drug therapy is particularly important if it includes cardioactive drugs, because these may interact with general anaesthetics that cause vasodilation and mild myocardial depression. Occasionally severe cardiovascular depression occurs under general anaesthesia from these combined effects. Previous anaesthetic problems may be known by the patient and must be sought. Some serious and potentially fatal anaesthetic diseases, such as malignant hyperthermia, are familial, and death under anaesthesia of a family member may indicate the presence of this disease. Such patients may wear Medic-Alert bracelets.

Examination

Airway and teeth should be examined, along with a general examination. The airway is fundamental to safe anaesthesia and must be kept patent at all times. It is very difficult to predict the ease of managing the airway. Anaesthetists try to assess which patients may have a difficult airway and thereby anticipate any potential problems. There are variants of normal anatomy that make anaesthetists suspicious about the airway; these include:

- short immobile neck
- buck teeth
- poor mouth opening
- recessive jaw, and
- an inability to sublux the lower incisors beyond the upper incisors.

24

Medical diseases can cause airway problems and these include:

- thyroid enlargement
- tumours of the head and neck, and
- musculoskeletal problems, such as ankylosing spondylitis and rheumatoid arthritis.

Loose teeth can be dislodged and broken and may be inhaled into the lungs.

Investigations

An acceptable haemoglobin for general anaesthesia is > 10.0 g/dl. Anaemia should be investigated to find its cause. Electrolyte disorders, such as hypokalaemia, should be corrected as general anaesthesia may otherwise be complicated by arrhythmias, prolongation of action of competitive neuromuscular relaxant drugs, decreased inotropism of the heart, and even respiratory muscle weakness after surgery.

Consent

Consent from the patient must be obtained.

Premedication

After assessment the anaesthetist will make a decision about the use of premedication. The reasons for premedication are shown in Box 5.3.

Usually oral sedative drugs are used. Topical EMLA cream can be used to prevent the pain of venepuncture. This eutectic mixture

---

Box 5.3 Reasons for premedication

- Relief of anxiety
- Antisialogogue
- Analgesia
- Antiemesis
- Amnesia
- Decreased gastric acidity
- Part of anaesthetic technique
- Prevent unwanted surgical responses – oculocardiac reflex
- Prevent pain of venepuncture

---

of prilocaine and lignocaine needs to be applied to the skin over the vein at least 1 hour before needle insertion.

All general anaesthetics have the same components. Following preoperative assessment and premedication, anaesthesia is induced, maintained, reversed, and finally postoperative care is given. The objectives of general anaesthesia for eye surgery are shown in Box 5.4.

Box 5.4 Objectives of general anaesthesia for eye surgery

- Immobile patient
- Airway control – proximity of surgeon
- Reduction of intraocular pressure
    avoid hypoxaemia
    avoid hypercarbia
    prevent hypertension
    prevent raised venous pressure – no coughing, straining, vomiting
    specific anaesthetic drugs contraindicated – ketamine, suxamethonium

---

Fluctuations in blood pressure during anaesthesia and surgery are important, because an abrupt increase when the globe is opened can result in iris prolapse and expulsive vitreous haemorrhage.

Airway

Control of the airway is crucial because of the proximity of the surgeon, and it is usually secured with either a laryngeal mask or a tracheal tube. The tracheal tube protects the airway from regurgitation of gastric contents, whereas the laryngeal mask does not. The tracheal tube is inserted with the aid of muscle relaxants which are of two types: competitive or non-competitive (depolarising). Depolarising agents, such as suxamethonium, work rapidly, last about 5 minutes, and are often used for emergency patients. Suxamethonium has many side effects, including raised intraocular pressure, bradycardia and anaphylaxis. It is responsible for the myalgia that patients often complain of postoperatively. Competitive agents have a slower onset of action, last about 30 minutes, and need to be reversed at the end of surgery. The patient may breathe spontaneously throughout the operation, or the lungs may be ventilated. The choice is often based on the personal preference of the anaesthetist. Better control of arterial and venous pressures can be achieved with a ventilated patient.

Emergency general anaesthesia

Emergency general anaesthesia is complicated by many factors, but the most important is that of the full stomach. After trauma, gastric emptying is delayed, and anaesthesia is complicated by the risk of vomiting, and the regurgitation of gastric contents, with subsequent aspiration into the lungs. Vomiting at induction of anaesthesia is particularly dangerous as the airway may be compromised. The techniques to deal with the problem are shown in Box 5.5.

Box 5.5 Management of tracheal intubation when risk of aspiration

- Empty stomach – nasogastric tube, metoclopramide
- Neutralise remaining stomach contents – antacids, H_2 antagonists prevent acid secretion
- Stop CNS-induced vomiting – use phenothiazines, avoid opiates
- Correct anaesthetic technique
      rapid sequence induction
      preoxygenation, cricoid pressure, tracheal intubation

The "at risk" patient is preoxygenated with 100% oxygen for 3 minutes to ensure that the lungs contain only oxygen and carbon dioxide, i.e. the lungs are denitrogenated. This provides a greater reservoir of oxygen to be taken up by the body and, in theory, there will be at least 5 minutes before oxygen needs to be given to the patient. Cricoid pressure is the application of pressure to the cricoid cartilage in the neck. This compresses the oesophagus against the vertebral column and stops the passive regurgitation of gastric contents into the pharynx and so protects the lungs. All emergency anaesthesia requires the trachea to be intubated; the cuff of the tracheal tube stops pharyngeal, gastric, and oesophageal debris entering the trachea.

6: Monitoring during surgery

Full monitoring of the patient under regional or general anaesthesia is mandatory. There are three basic requirements of monitoring (Box 6.1).

Box 6.1 Anaesthetic monitoring requirements

- Presence of trained anaesthetist/suitably qualified practitioner
- Checking and monitoring of equipment
- Patient monitoring
    clinical
    technical

Who should monitor the patient?

Regional anaesthesia for eye surgery is increasingly being undertaken by anaesthetists. This is a recent development over the past decade. When an anaesthetist performs the eye block, the responsibility for the patient lies with that anaesthetist. Some surgeons undertake their own regional anaesthesia and take responsibility for the intraoperative care of the patient. This practice is unsafe unless it is carried out in an operating theatre where there is immediate access to anaesthetic help. In these circumstances, it is a minimal requirement that a trained operating department practitioner checks the oxygen supply and anaesthetic equipment, and monitors the patient throughout the operation. Audible alarms are recommended. An intravenous cannula must be inserted before surgery takes place.

An anaesthetist must monitor all patients undergoing general anaesthesia, and that anaesthetist must be present and vigilant throughout the operation and must check all the equipment in use. The function and use of the oxygen supply devices (cylinders and/or pipelines) must be understood by all theatre personnel and oxygen failure alarms must be in working order.

Patient monitoring

It is essential to observe the patient's colour, chest movement, respiration, and heart rate, and to look for signs of sympathetic overactivity, such as sweating. Continuous monitoring of the circulatory and respiratory systems by means of appropriate equipment is also necessary. We recommend that eye anaesthesia is carried out with the use of the equipment listed in Box 6.2.

Box 6.2 Routine technical monitoring devices

- Cardiovascular
    electrocardiogram (for heart rate and arrhythmias)
    non-invasive arterial pressure
    oximeter
- Respiration
    respiratory rate
    end-tidal carbon dioxide concentration (general anaesthesia only)
    inspired oxygen concentration
- Muscle relaxation (general anaesthesia only)
    peripheral nerve stimulator

Problems may occur when the eye patient is being monitored. A fully draped patient is difficult to observe and it is important to be able to see clearly some part of the patient, such as an arm or a foot. Monitoring the patient's blood pressure during surgery under local anaesthesia can cause anxiety and even pain, and this may cause the patient to move unexpectedly. The cuff should be connected, but only inflated if necessary, and only after the patient has been warned of what is about to happen.

The staff responsible for monitoring the patient must understand the electrocardiogram. Abnormal rhythms should be identified and the designated anaesthetist called. Bradycardia is the most common abnormality seen and usually results from the oculocardiac reflex. If the heart rate decreases by 20%, the surgeon must stop all traction on the eye and the anaesthetist must be called. The anaesthetist must attend if the patient becomes extremely anxious or unco-operative during the procedure. This may indicate an acute medical emergency, such as difficulty in breathing from heart failure. Prolonged operations can result in hypothermia and occasionally temperature monitoring is necessary.

Essential monitoring adds to the safety of operations under general anaesthesia, but the perfect monitoring device is not available. The ability to monitor the depth of anaesthesia would enable the anaesthetist to avoid the problem of patient awareness, that can occur when minimal general anaesthesia is used in elderly frail patients.

7: The paediatric patient

Children merit special consideration. Young children are easily frightened, often distressed by pain, and may not understand the surgery. Infants and young children are nearly always accompanied by at least one adult who needs an explanation of the nature of the surgery and anaesthesia.

Surgery and anaesthesia are specialised in this group of patients. A surgical unit looking after children needs more space, great flexibility and careful design, and the medical and nursing care must be orientated to the children. Nurses should be trained specifically for paediatric care, and the ophthalmologists, anaesthetists, and paediatricians must work closely together to provide the appropriate expertise (Box 7.1).

Box 7.1 Requirements for paediatric patients

- Patient and parental education
- Environment – appropriate decor, facilities for parents to stay with patient, play area
- Medical care – specialist ophthalmologist, access to paediatricians
- Nursing care – paediatric trained staff
- Operating lists – ideally, specific paediatric lists
- Recovery facilities – ideally, children with own recovery area separated from adults, parental visiting encouraged

---

Eye surgery in children

Approximately 10% of eye operations are undertaken in children. There are two main indications:

- Examination and minor operative procedures (e.g. eyelid surgery) on the eye. These rarely require general anaesthesia in an adult, but in children general anaesthesia is necessary to ensure immobility and co-operation.

- To improve future vision or vision-related tasks. For example, in squint surgery and treatment for congenital cataract, the aim is to facilitate development of the visual system.

The decision to operate

The principles behind the decision to operate are outlined in Chapter 1. In paediatric ophthalmology it is of paramount importance to discuss with the parents or guardians the expectations and consequences of the surgery, so that they are able to make an informed decision on behalf of their child. In many instances there are unrealistic expectations of surgery and it is important to discuss how it contributes to the treatment required to develop the child's visual potential fully. For example, the infant with squint may need glasses, eye patches, and perhaps further surgery during the management of the problem.

Preoperative assessment in children

It is important for the child to be comfortable in, and preferably familiar with, the pre- and postoperative environment. To allay anxiety it can be useful to carry out the preoperative assessment in the postoperative area. Children with eye problems are more likely to have other systemic diseases, and some of these are relevant to anaesthesia. Children with squints, for example, are claimed to have a higher incidence of malignant hyperthermia (see Chapter 8).

Anaesthesia

Premedication is used commonly in children to allay anxiety and provide sedation. Midazolam syrup 0.5 mg/kg can be administered orally 20 minutes before induction of anaesthesia. Some anaesthetists give oral atropine 0.02 mg/kg with the premedication to prevent intraoperative bradycardia resulting from the oculocardiac reflex, although most now give the drug intravenously as its action is more predictable by this route. EMLA cream is used to prevent needle pain and is applied 1 hour before anaesthesia.

Most centres now allow children to eat solid food up to 4 hours before, and to drink clear fluids up to 2 hours before surgery. Anaesthesia is usually induced intravenously but some children prefer an inhalational technique. Suitably informed and sensible parents are encouraged to be with the child in the anaesthetic room, but an especially anxious parent may not be particularly helpful, and the final decision as to whether a parent is allowed to stay in the anaesthetic room lies with the anaesthetist.

The specific problems of paediatric anaesthesia are shown in Box 7.2.

Box 7.2 Anaesthetic paediatric problems

- Different anatomy and physiology compared with an adult
- Different pharmacological responses compared with an adult
- Psychological preparation of child and family
- Associated diseases
- Difficulty with regional anaesthetic techniques
- Oculocardiac reflex
- Oculorespiratory reflex
- Postoperative nausea and vomiting
- Postoperative analgesia

The oculocardiac reflex is seen frequently in strabismus surgery and is triggered by pressure on the globe and traction on the orbital muscles. The reflex has an afferent pathway via the short and long ciliary nerves, part of the ophthalmic branch of the fifth cranial nerve that synapses in the trigeminal nucleus in the ventral surface of the pons in the brainstem. The efferent pathway is in the vagus nerve, stimulation of which causes bradycardia. Any cardiac arrhythmia can be induced by this reflex and it may occur in 90% of unpremedicated children. It is prevented and treated by anticholinergic drugs such as glycopyrrolate and atropine.

The oculorespiratory reflex has a similar afferent pathway to the oculocardiac reflex and the efferent limb terminates in the respiratory centre. The result is shallow breathing, or apnoea, in spontaneously breathing patients.

Vomiting is common after squint surgery and many anaesthetists try to prevent it by using antiemetics prophylactically. Unfortunately, the incidence of vomiting declines little, whatever is tried, which is frustrating for both patients and staff.

Postoperative analgesia is usually managed by simple analgesics; oral paracetamol 15 mg/kg is often sufficient.

Postoperative care of children

It may be alarming for parents of very young children and infants to nurse a child after eye surgery, because tears can appear blood-stained and they are afraid that the child will rub his or her eye. It is important that these fears are allayed. It is most unlikely that the child will injure the eye by rubbing and tears are always blood-stained after eye operations. On the other hand, robust activity and direct injury to the eye should be prevented in the immediate postoperative period. The duration of this period will vary with the surgery.

It is important to inform the parents or guardian about the likely postoperative course on discharge from hospital, and to give appropriate contact numbers (Box 7.3).

Box 7.3 Information required on discharge from hospital

- Surgical information
    name of procedure
    name of consultant
    details of discharge medication
    need for eye patch
- The next 24 hours
    when child can eat or drink
    postoperative analgesia prescribed
    information about postoperative symptoms – transient double vision, red eye
- Next hospital appointment – date, time, place, and with whom
- Emergency contact numbers
- Telephone number for advice

Sometimes an eye dressing (eye patch) will be required after surgery; it is important for the parents or guardian to know whether they should replace the patch in the immediate postoperative period should it be removed by the child.

8: Perioperative crises

Sudden, life-threatening complications occur rarely, but must be recognised and treated appropriately.

Patients unable to cope with surgery under regional anaesthesia

Patients can suffer from claustrophobia under surgical drapes. It must be remembered, however, that all problems are not psychological. Problems should be considered in the ways shown in Box 8.1.

Box 8.1 Problems under regional anaesthesia

- Patient factors – psychological
- Surgical factors – pain, prolonged surgery
- Medical factors – congestive heart failure, lung disease
- Anaesthetic factors – inadvertent intravascular injection, brainstem anaesthesia

---

Anaphylactic reactions

Minor allergic reactions as a result of drug administration are not uncommon. Major reactions, caused by drugs administered in general anaesthesia (especially muscle relaxants), or local anaesthetic drugs, are fortunately rare. An increasingly recognised cause of anaphylaxis is latex allergy which starts 30–60 min after surgery. The signs of anaphylaxis are shown in Box 8.2.

Management of anaphylaxis

This should be considered in two parts: immediate (Box 8.3) and secondary (Box 8.4).

The following guidelines assume a patient of 70 kg weight in whom the diagnosis of anaphylaxis is obvious. Administration of intravenous adrenaline is a priority.

Box 8.2 Signs of anaphylaxis

- Pruritis
- Erythema
- Nausea, vomiting, and diarrhoea
- Angio-oedema
- Laryngeal oedema with stridor
- Bronchospasm and wheeze
- Hypotension
- Cardiovascular collapse
- Disseminated intravascular coagulation
- Sudden death

Box 8.3 Immediate management of anaphylaxis

- Call for help
- Stop suspected drug, if possible
- Stop surgery and anaesthesia
- Maintain airway
- **Give 100% oxygen** – consider tracheal intubation and ventilation
- **Intravenous adrenaline** in aliquots of 0.5–1.0 ml of 1:10 000
- **Intravascular fluid replacement** by colloid, e.g. haemaccel 10 ml/kg bolus
- Consider cardiopulmonary resuscitation

Box 8.4 Secondary management of anaphylaxis

- Adrenaline-resistant bronchospasm – intravenous aminophylline 4–8 mg/kg over 20 min
- Consider intravenous hydrocortisone 300 mg or methylprednisolone 2 g
- Consider antihistamines – intravenous chlorpheniramine 20 mg over 20 min
- Consider administering intravenous sodium bicarbonate
- Catecholamine infusions – intravenous adrenaline 5 mg in 500 ml at rate of 10–85 ml/h
- Consider that a coagulopathy may be present – do a clotting screen
- Arterial gas analysis

In the secondary management of anaphylaxis, it is important to remember that intensive care facilities are needed.

After severe reactions the patient must be investigated. Blood tests are taken initially with serial samples at 6 and 24 hours for serum tryptase (a neutral protease released from mast cells), complement activation, and IgE antibody concentrations. These will confirm that an anaphylactic reaction has occurred, but will not identify the agent.

A full medical history must be taken and after 4 weeks the patient referred for "skin prick" tests to a clinical immunologist. The incident must be reported to the Committee on Safety of Medicines and the patient should be advised to wear a Medic-Alert bracelet. The patient's general practitioner should be informed.

Cardiac arrest

The causes of cardiac arrest both within and outside the operating theatre can be classified under three headings:

- Medical factors – cardiac disease, electrolyte disturbances
- Surgical factors – asystole from reflexes like the oculocardiac reflex, accidental intravenous injection of local anaesthetics
- Anaesthetic factors – failure to secure the airway, disconnection of the anaesthetic circuit, pneumothorax, drugs.

All medical staff must be continuously trained in the management of cardiac arrest; they must be able to use a defibrillator, and know where it is kept. Basic and Advanced Life Support management algorithms are shown in Box 8.5 and 8.6 respectively.

Following Basic Life Support, Advanced Life Support must be instigated.

In monitored patients, clinical and electrocardiographic detection of cardiac arrest should be nearly simultaneous. In these situations a precordial thump can be used. The first three defibrillation shocks (200 J, 200 J, 360 J) should be given within 60 seconds. The dose of adrenaline used is 1 mg (10 ml 1:10 000).

Malignant hyperthermia

This is a rare complication of general anaesthesia which results in an abnormal increase in muscle metabolism in

Box 8.5 Algorithm for Basic Life Support (BLS)

- Check responsiveness – shake and shout
- Open airway – head tilt/chin lift
- Check breathing – look, listen, feel
    If patient is breathing, place in recovery position
    If patient is not breathing, give two effective breaths (mouth to mouth/nose)
- Assess for 10 seconds only – is there a circulation?
    If circulation present – continue rescue breathing, check circulation every minute
    No circulation – compress chest at 100/min (ratio of 15 compressions: 2 breaths)
- Get help as soon as possible

Box 8.6 Algorithm for Advanced Life Support (ALS)

- BLS algorithm, if appropriate
- Precordial thump, if appropriate
- Attach monitor/defibrillator
- Assess rhythm and check pulse
    If VT/VF – defibrillate × 3 as necessary, CPR 1 min and assess rhythm
    If non VF/VT – up to 3 min CPR and assess rhythm
- During CPR if not already undertaken
    Check electrode/paddle positions and contact
    Attempt/verify tracheal intubation and i.v. access
- Give adrenaline every 3 min
- Correct reversible causes
- Consider: buffers, antiarrhythmics, atropine (pacing – medical team input)
- Potentially reversible causes
    Hypoxaemia
    Hypovolaemia
    Hyper/hypokalaemia and metabolic disorders
    Hypothermia
    Tension pneumothorax
    Tamponade
    Toxic/therapeutic disturbances – drugs
    Thromboembolic/mechanical obstruction to circulation

response to the volatile anaesthetic agents or the muscle relaxant suxamethonium. The incidence varies, but is cited as between 1:10 000 and 1:50 000 anaesthetics. It is more common in children and young male adults, and in those with congenital musculoskeletal disorders. There is often a family history of unexpected death, or problems associated with general anaesthesia, and it is inherited as an autosomal dominant condition.

The problem can occur either at the start of, or during maintenance of, general anaesthesia. Patients can develop masseter spasm after suxamethonium on induction of anaesthesia. Common presenting signs are tachycardia, tachypnoea, cyanosis, muscle stiffness, and pyrexia. Metabolic changes include acidosis, raised carbon dioxide production, and hyperkalaemia.

Management is by supportive measures to treat the acidosis and hyperkalaemia, and specifically by giving dantrolene, which must be available in every theatre. Tragically, deaths under general anaesthesia still occur from failure to recognise the onset of the condition, despite the availability of dantrolene.

Brainstem anaesthesia

If a local anaesthetic drug is inadvertently injected into the cerebrospinal fluid during administration of a retrobulbar block, brainstem anaesthesia can result. This rare, but potentially fatal, complication will cause respiratory arrest and blockade of the sympathetic nervous system with consequent bradycardia and hypotension. The patient's breathing will have to be supported by artificial ventilation until the effects of the local anaesthetic wear off.

Onset of brainstem anaesthesia occurs within minutes and ventilation may have to be assisted for up to 2 hours. The patient remains aware, despite the paralysis, and sedation must be provided.

Crises caused by orbital injections for regional anaesthesia

The main sign of **globe perforation** is hypotony. The surgery must be postponed and a retinal examination performed to identify and treat with laser or prophylactic cryotherapy any entry or exit wounds.

Retrobulbar haemorrhage caused by needle trauma to

arteries or veins within the orbit may need lateral canthotomy to reduce intraorbital pressure and prevent central retinal artery occlusion. Surgery is postponed and rescheduled for general or topical anaesthesia at a later date.

40

9: Recovery unit

After regional anaesthesia, recovery facilities are not usually required. However, after general anaesthesia, the awakening patient is routinely transferred to the recovery unit on completion of surgery. Trained staff care for the patient on a "one to one" basis until the effects of anaesthesia have worn off sufficiently for care to be continued in the ward. Whilst in the unit, the patient remains the responsibility of the anaesthetist and the surgeon, both of whom must be available to deal with complications should they arise.

The objectives of recovery room care are shown in Box 9.1.

Box 9.1 Objectives of the recovery unit

- Clinical observation
- Assessment of conscious level
- Essential monitoring (readings can be at 15 min intervals) – pulse rate, blood pressure, respiration, oxygen saturation, temperature
- Airway management
- Oxygen therapy
- Pain control
- Prevention and treatment of nausea and vomiting
- Temperature control
- Avoidance of shivering
- Intravenous fluid management

The management of the airway is the most important immediate goal. Failure to secure a patent airway can lead to cyanosis, hypoxaemia, and hypercarbia. Cyanosis usually occurs because of failure to oxygenate the patient, although it can result from depression of the cardiovascular system.

Oxygen therapy is given routinely after general anaesthesia, normally via a "variable performance" face mask such as a Hudson mask: 4 litres/min provides about 40% inspired oxygen and this is used commonly. Nasal cannulae are occasionally used, but are less effective. Oxygen saturation is monitored continuously by an oximeter attached to the finger. This device measures the percentage of haemoglobin that is saturated with oxygen, and normal values are 95–97%. Saturations below 90% are regarded as unsafe and represent inadequate tissue perfusion with oxygen. The reading can be interfered with by excessive patient movement, a cold periphery, venous congestion, nail polish, false nails and, rarely, by drugs.

Common causes of hypoxaemia immediately after surgery are shown in Box 9.2. The usual cause is airway obstruction, but hypoventilation resulting from the effects of anaesthesia and muscle relaxants can occur. Shivering, especially after surgery in a cold theatre, leads to an increased oxygen consumption.

Box 9.2 Common causes of immediate postoperative hypoxaemia

- Hypoventilation
    airway obstruction
    central respiratory depression
    respiratory muscle weakness
- Increased oxygen consumption
    shivering
- Lung ventilation/perfusion mismatch
- Low oxygen content of blood
    low cardiac output
    low haemoglobin level

Complications in the recovery room

Airway obstruction

During emergence from anaesthesia, patients have incomplete control of the tongue, as well as suppressed laryngeal and pharyngeal reflexes, and active maintenance of the airway is required to prevent hypoxaemia. This is why patients are normally managed in the left lateral or "recovery position" after anaesthesia (which makes intubation of the trachea easier for the anaesthetist if difficulties arise). After eye surgery patients are positioned with the operative site upwards to prevent pressure on the operated eye and this makes attention to the airway even more critical.

Box 9.3 Signs of airway obstruction

- "See-saw" pattern of respiration
- Tachypnoea
- Cyanosis
- Tachycardia
- Hypertension
- Arrhythmias
- Anxiety
- Sweating
- Low oxygen saturation

The signs of airway obstruction in a patient are listed in Box 9.3. This complication arises most commonly from obstruction by the tongue, but can occasionally be due to laryngeal spasm or laryngeal oedema.

Airway obstruction is treated by extension of the neck, jaw thrust, and insertion of an oropharyngeal airway to ensure airway patency. Laryngeal spasm results from spasm of the vocal cords and causes postoperative stridor. It is commonly a response to airway stimulation in a lightly anaesthetised patient. It can be frightening and lead to severe hypoxaemia and even pulmonary oedema. Administering oxygen and ensuring a patent airway usually leads to its swift resolution. Occasionally the anaesthetist will need to intubate the trachea to ensure oxygenation. Laryngeal oedema is treated by intravenous dexamethasone 8 mg.

Failure to breathe

Failure to breathe at the end of anaesthesia has many possible causes and these are listed in Box 9.4.

The most common cause is central nervous system depression from injudicious opiate usage. A peripheral nerve stimulator is necessary to differentiate between central and peripheral causes.

Nausea and vomiting

Nausea and vomiting are unpleasant side effects of anaesthesia. Associated factors are listed in Box 9.5.

Box 9.4 Causes of failure to breathe at the end of anaesthesia

- Central nervous system
    drug depression – particularly opiates, inhalational agents
    decreased respiratory drive – hypocapnia
    central nervous system damage
- Peripheral
    failure of normal neuromuscular transmission
- Hypothermia
- Drug interactions
- Electrolyte disorders – hypokalaemia
- Undiagnosed skeletal muscle disorders – myasthenia gravis

Box 9.5 Factors associated with nausea and vomiting

- Patient predisposition
    age, sex, obesity
    history of motion sickness and previous postoperative
    vomiting
    pain, food ingestion
- Surgical factors
    type of surgery, emergency or elective
- Anaesthetic factors
    type and duration of anaesthesia
    experience of anaesthetist
- Postoperative factors
    pain
    hypotension
    hypoxaemia
    patient movement
    first intake of fluids/food
    early mobilisation

Delayed awakening

Failure to recover full consciousness after anaesthesia is cause for great concern. The most common reasons are drug related, but hypothermia, hypoglycaemia, hyponatraemia, and hypothyroidism must be considered (Box 9.6).

Box 9.6 Causes of delayed recovery from anaesthesia

- Hypoxaemia
- Hypocapnia
- Residual anaesthesia, usually volatile agents
- Drugs – opiates
- Emergence delirium – ketamine, scopolamine, atropine
- Neurological problems
- Surgical
- Metabolic – hypoglycaemia, hyponatraemia
- Medical – hypothyroidism
- Sepsis
- Hypothermia

Shivering

Shivering is common after anaesthesia but is not obviously related to a low core temperature in the patient. The main deleterious effect is an increase in oxygen consumption and it should be treated promptly, especially in the elderly. Treatment should be prophylactic and normothermia maintained if possible. The judicious use of doxapram and pethidine helps to control shivering when it occurs.

Temperature disturbances

A decrease in body temperature is the inevitable consequence of general anaesthesia. Factors predisposing to hypothermia include a cool theatre, patient's age, duration of surgery, concomitant disease, cold intravenous fluids, and drugs. The sequelae include shivering, impaired platelet aggregation, and decreased drug metabolism. Ideally, theatre temperature should be maintained at 24°C, inspired anaesthetic gases humidified, intravenous fluids warmed, and skin surfaces warmed by means of passive insulation, or actively (water blanket, radiant heater, forced air warmer) in an attempt to prevent hypothermia.

Hyperthermia after anaesthesia is rare, and infection is the most common cause. Drugs such as atropine in large doses prevent sweating and rarely may cause a rise in temperature.

Discharge from recovery unit

Criteria for discharge from the recovery room to the ward are becoming increasingly common and important, and are listed in Box 9.7. The patient should be transferred to the ward in a stable condition and relevant information should be communicated carefully and fully to the ward staff.

Box 9.7 Typical criteria for recovery unit discharge

- No surgical complications
- Patient awake and responding appropriately to commands
- Upper airway patent and reflexes present
- Breathing satisfactory
- Cardiovascular stability
- Pain control adequate
- No vomiting
- Transfer of appropriate information to ward staff

10: Fitness for hospital discharge

Guidelines for discharge

Hospital discharge, especially after uncomplicated day surgery, requires adequate recovery from anaesthesia. Most units have specific guidelines for discharge after general anaesthesia (Box 10.1), and these may be quantified by using scoring systems. A typical discharge scoring system is shown in Appendix D at the end of the book.

Box 10.1 Discharge criteria after eye surgery under general anaesthesia

- Stable vital signs (heart rate, blood pressure, breathing) for 1 hour
- No evidence of respiratory depression
- Patients must be
    orientated in person, place, time, or to their preoperative mental status
    able to drink oral fluids
    able to dress themselves (consistent with their preoperative state)
    able to walk (consistent with their preoperative state)
    able to urinate
- Patients must have no nausea or vomiting
- Patients must have minimal pain and bleeding
- A responsible fit adult must be able to escort them home and stay with them for 6 hours and preferably overnight
- Patients must have written instructions for postoperative care including contact numbers for eye clinic, on-call eye doctors, and general practitioner

---

Elderly men are notoriously unreliable at urinating on demand and this may prevent discharge from hospital. To avoid unnecessary admissions, it is wise to anaesthetise elderly people early in the day.

Eye operations using regional anaesthesia require less stringent guidance for discharge. It is reasonable for patients to be allowed home within 1 hour of surgery provided that all the criteria in Box 10.2 are met.

Box 10.2 Guidelines for discharge home after eye surgery under regional anaesthesia

- Patients must be orientated to their preoperative state
- Patients who are unable to see with the operated eye covered must have an escort until the dressing can be removed
- The eye dressing should be comfortable
- There should be no excessive pain or bleeding
- Pre-arranged transport to the patient's home should be used for all major procedures
- Patients should have access to a telephone at home
- Patients must have written instructions for pain relief, anticipated postoperative course and emergency contact numbers (see Appendix E)

Pain relief

Adequate pain relief is an important aspect of rapid discharge from hospital and, if poorly managed, will undermine the patient's confidence in the outcome of the surgical procedure. Fortunately, postoperative pain is not a common feature of eye surgery. However, significant pain can be anticipated after corneal surgery and after procedures associated with a marked inflammatory response within the orbit. Patients undergoing any of the operations in Box 10.3 should be warned to expect pain after surgery and should be discharged home with adequate analgesia for the immediate postoperative period.

After routine eye surgery, the patient should be advised to take simple medication for postoperative discomfort, as they would for a headache. Normally this would be a drug such as paracetamol (8 tablets per day, maximum adult dose – 4 g). If more severe pain is anticipated, non-steroidal anti-inflammatory drugs (NSAIDs), such as diclofenac, may be prescribed and are more effective than simple analgesics. However, these drugs are associated with important side effects (Box 10.4) and should be used with caution in elderly patients.

Box 10.3 Eye surgery with significant postoperative pain

- Corneal surgery
    pterygium excision
    photorefractive keratectomy
    inadvertent corneal abrasion
- Vitreoretinal procedures
- Complex squint surgery
- Orbital procedures

Box 10.4 Important side effects of NSAIDs

- Renal impairment
- Gastric ulceration
- Decreased platelet aggregation
- Drug interactions (e.g. serum potassium with diuretic use)
- Hypersensitivity

Follow-up arrangements

It is important that the patient, and their health team, are clear about the pattern of continuing care both in the immediate and long term. In most cases a follow-up appointment with the eye team will be the next step. Until that appointment, the patient needs to know what to expect and what needs to be done with eye dressings and medications. This is best achieved by discussion with the day unit team and reinforced with written advice.

Special discharge and transport arrangements may be needed for those living alone or in sheltered or residential accommodation, and these must be made in advance of the admission.

It is important that patients who have undergone general anaesthesia are told to abstain from drinking alcohol, driving a car, riding a bicycle or operating machinery for at least 24 hours.

It is useful to have a checklist of arrangements to be made before discharge (Box 10.5).

Box 10.5 Discharge checklist

- Outpatient appointment, or clear instructions about follow-up
- Advice on instilling eye medication
- Advice on the eye dressing (e.g. that it is to remain in place until removed by the nurse the following morning)
- Analgesia
- Contact telephone numbers and emergency facilities
- Intravenous cannula removed
- Discharge letter given to patient

11: Complications in the community

A major concern following day-stay surgery is that early complications may be missed. Important signs indicating postoperative complications can be overlooked because the patient is at home. This possibility can be greatly decreased by confining day-stay surgery to procedures in which complications are unlikely to occur. However, with time, guidelines for day-stay surgery will be relaxed, increasing the risk of complications being diagnosed too late.

It is sensible to prepare the patient to expect certain symptoms after surgery and to look out for others. Patients should telephone the unit if these latter symptoms occur or, in some instances, return to hospital promptly. Generally, the patient should seek help if any significant new symptom occurs within two weeks after surgery and before the first clinic visit. Most general practitioners feel unable to diagnose and treat postoperative eye problems, so symptomatic patients must be referred directly back to the ophthalmologist.

In this chapter simple guidance is given about how to manage expected postoperative symptoms and how to distinguish those that may indicate the development of complications.

Symptoms in the first 24 hours

Pain

Once anaesthesia has worn off, most patients experience discomfort at the site of the operation. Patients should expect their pain to be relieved by simple analgesics, such as paracetamol, and the discomfort should not be severe enough to interrupt sleep.

Increasing severity of pain in the first 24 hours is unusual and may indicate a serious complication (Box 11.1). The patient in severe pain must contact the eye unit and be prepared to attend for examination. Intraocular infection is the most serious complication of eye surgery. It may destroy vision and must be diagnosed and treated promptly.

Box 11.1 Causes and treatment of increasing postoperative eye pain

- Infection – culture organism from swabs and prescribe antibiotics either drops, or systemic, depending on the site of infection
- Inflammation – provide pupillary dilation after intraocular surgery and increase the frequency of steroid drops and/or ointment
- Raised eye pressure – pressure reduction by appropriate drops or oral medication, occasionally surgical intervention
- Corneal abrasion – eye closed, use pad, with daily examination until healing has occurred

---

Double vision

After squint surgery patients may experience double vision. The brain takes time to become accustomed to the new eye position and symptoms often settle within a few days, but occasionally it can take weeks. The patient should inform the eye unit of troublesome double vision, as specific exercises can be sometimes recommended to help resolve the problem.

Following local anaesthetic injections around the globe of the eye, there may be double vision for a day or so. This usually recovers spontaneously.

Changes in hue after cataract surgery

A rose-tinted hue is often reported after cataract surgery in patients who had dense yellowing of the natural lens. This is not significant and adjustment usually occurs within a few days.

Symptoms related to general anaesthesia

Nearly all the drugs given in general anaesthesia are metabolised and excreted within 24 hours of the operation. Patients often complain of a sore throat which settles spontaneously; this is caused by the tracheal tube. Patients who have received the muscle relaxant, suxamethonium, may complain of aching muscles resulting from the muscle fasciculations caused by the drug. Nausea and vomiting after anaesthesia should be controlled before discharge. Patients should not make major decisions for 24 hours after anaesthesia. Some drugs given in anaesthesia can cause urinary retention and patients should be aware of this possibility.

Symptoms arising in the first two weeks

It is usual for postoperative symptoms to be worst on the first postoperative day and to improve gradually over subsequent weeks. A sudden reversal of improvement is a bad sign.

Decreased vision/increased pain

An abrupt decrease in acuity or increase in pain following cataract surgery can indicate intraocular infection, and the patient must return immediately to hospital. Other causes of reduced vision, such as changes in the depth of the anterior chamber following trabeculectomy, often resolve without an adverse outcome.

Pain may indicate suture-related problems, abnormally high intraocular pressure, increased inflammation, or an ocular surface abnormality. An eye examination is necessary to determine the cause and appropriate management.

Increasing redness around the eye

Although some hyperaemia or bruising is anticipated, especially following lid surgery and injections around the eye, increasing redness postoperatively may indicate allergy to the prescribed, postoperative antibiotic drops. If this is suspected, the drops should be stopped and the hospital's advice sought about whether an alternative should be used.

Symptoms following mild trauma

Although patients are asked to avoid any damage to the eye after intraocular surgery, it is not uncommon for minor trauma to cause wound rupture or iris prolapse within the first two weeks. These complications may be asymptomatic but can cause increased watering, redness, discharge, pain, and blurred vision. Patients **must** return to the eye unit if any of these symptoms occur within two weeks of surgery, especially after minor trauma.

Delayed symptoms related to the anaesthesia

The intravenous cannula can cause thrombosis of the vein into which it was inserted. Although this may be painful, it is almost invariably without sequelae. Long-term complications are rare but pain in the leg or calf may indicate a deep vein thrombosis. Similarly, the sudden onset of sharp chest pain may indicate pulmonary embolism secondary to deep vein thrombosis. Medical advice must be sought as a matter of urgency in these circumstances.

12: Outpatient investigations and surgery

Outpatient ophthalmology now encompasses many procedures once confined to the operating theatre (Box 12.1) and it is likely that the trend will continue. Currently, there are no specific guidelines on anaesthetic monitoring in ophthalmic outpatients. In this chapter, we suggest a sensible approach to safe practice in the outpatient clinic.

Box 12.1 Ophthalmic outpatient procedures

- Laser surgery
  retinal laser photocoagulation
  Nd YAG laser procedures e.g. capsulotomy, iridotomy
  ciliary body ablation
- Cryotherapy
- Periocular and intraocular injections and biopsies
- Suture removal
- Suture adjustment following corneal and squint surgery
- Lid surgery
  minor, as in chalazion incision and curettage
  major, as in entropion repair

Fainting in the outpatient clinic

It is not uncommon for patients to faint in the ophthalmic outpatient clinic. Although it is usually associated with minor procedures such as removal of a corneal foreign body, a vasovagal reflex may be provoked by eye examination alone. It is impractical and unnecessary to monitor all minor procedures, but it is important that outpatient staff are alerted to this common reaction, and that they recognise the early signs and symptoms (sweating, pallor, vomiting, dizziness, slurred speech, unsteady gait, unconsciousness, hypotension, bradycardia). They must be able to prevent an unconscious patient being hurt when falling to the floor. Outpatient furniture and equipment should be moved in an emergency. Therefore, all heavy apparatus must be on wheels, especially when it is in a confined area. Instruction in basic cardiac resuscitation must be given to eye clinic staff on a regular basis, and there must be access to life-support equipment within the department (Box 12.2).

Box 12.2 Essential resuscitation equipment

- Intravenous cannulae, infusion sets and fluids – 0.9% sodium chloride, haemaccel
- Defibrillator and electrocardiograph
- Drugs – box containing
    4 ampoules 10 ml adrenaline 1:10 000
    1 ampoule 10 ml atropine 3 mg
    2 ampoules 10 ml aminophylline 250 mg
    2 ampoules 2 ml diazepam 10 mg
    2 ampoules 20 ml glucose 20%
    3 ampoules 1 ml naloxone 0.4 mg
- Guedel airways – sizes 1,2,3,4
- Ambubag to provide assisted ventilation, via an oxygen supply
- Range of laryngoscopes, tracheal tubes and connectors

Life-threatening events in the outpatient clinic

These are normally either cardiac or respiratory in nature. High risk patients are those with a predisposing cardiac or respiratory problem, or those who are undergoing a painful or distressing procedure (Box 12.3). It is important that medically unstable patients are treated optimally before their outpatient procedure.

Box 12.3 Painful outpatient procedures

- Ciliary body ablation: cyclodiode, cycloYAG, cyclocryotherapy
- Panretinal photocoagulation under peribulbar or retrobulbar anaesthesia
- Intraocular injections and biopsies
- Major lid surgery

Fluorescein angiography

Retinal angiography with an intravenous solution of 20% sodium fluorescein is a common investigative procedure in ophthalmology outpatient departments. The most frequent serious side effect is bronchospasm, but more severe life-threatening reactions have been reported (myocardial infarction, hypertensive crisis, pulmonary oedema) with an incidence of up to six investigations in 1000. Written consent is mandatory and staff need to be trained to recognise problems and administer resuscitation appropriately.

Monitoring in ophthalmic outpatients

Patients undergoing surgery may receive regional anaesthesia for the procedure (see Chapter 4). The minimum requirement for monitoring has been discussed previously (see Chapter 6) and the same requirements should ideally be met in the outpatient clinic. There are very few ophthalmology outpatient departments with access to the necessary facilities and appropriately trained staff. It is accepted practice to agree monitoring guidelines locally between anaesthetic and ophthalmic surgical teams. The principle behind such guidelines must be to ensure the safety of the patient. In an outpatient department where monitoring is not possible, complex procedures must be performed in main theatres with appropriate anaesthetic cover.

Appendix A: Risks of eye surgery leaflet

Eye surgery carries minimal risk to the general well-being of the patient. Although it is one of the safest types of surgery, there are important complications that you should be aware of.

Risks of surgery within the eye

Surgery within the eye, e.g. cataract surgery, carries both surgical complications and anaesthetic risks. Technical surgical problems can cause minor complications at the time of surgery, or soon after, and occur with a frequency of up to four in a 100 operations. These usually resolve with good visual outcome, but perhaps delay recovery from surgery. Major problems during or following surgery within the eye (major haemorrhage or infection) are rare (one in a 1000) and may occur even in technically un-complicated surgery. The result may be a blind eye or severely impaired vision despite vigorous treatment.

Surgery to structures around the eye

Surgery to structures around the eye, e.g. squint surgery, has few ocular complications. Anaesthetic and technical problems may nevertheless arise and each operation must be discussed fully in terms of anticipated specific risks.

Risks of anaesthesia

Local anaesthesia

Local anaesthesia carries less risk to the general well-being of the patient, although one in 500 may experience an adverse reaction to the anaesthetic. A full recovery is expected. Risk to the eye from the local anaesthetic may also occur. Major complications (e.g. needle perforation of the globe) may result in blindness, but are rare (reported incidence one in a 1000 patients). Minor complications (temporary bruising, lid droop, muscle weakness) are short lived and full recovery is usual.

General anaesthesia

General anaesthesia also carries risks. Some, such as drug allergy, are exceedingly rare but potentially serious. In addition, you will be asked about problems with your general health, previous anaesthetics, and whether there is a family history of anaesthetic problems. This is to minimise risk. Minor complications (e.g. sore throat, nausea, and vomiting) occur more frequently, but are transient in nature, and you should feel normal within 24 hours.

Appendix B: Cataract surgery leaflet

Before the operation

You will be given a date and time to come to the pre-assessment clinic to review your general health and home circumstances and to take measurements of your eye. There will be an opportunity to discuss any worries or uncertainties that you may have with nurses and doctors involved with your operation.

On the day

It is important for you to follow the instructions about the food and drink allowed before your surgery so as not to delay the operation. After checking in, you will be prepared for surgery. Your clothes and belongings will be placed in a locker. A staff member will put drops in your eye to dilate the pupil and numb the surface of the eye. You will be transferred to the operating theatre suite and attached to monitors that measure blood pressure and heart beat patterns. In addition, a small needle will be inserted into an arm vein. These are routine precautions taken to ensure your safety during the operation.

Your anaesthetic will then be administered. If you are having a local anaesthetic, a small pressure ball may be placed over your eye after the insertion of the local anaesthetic drugs for a few minutes before the start of the surgery. With local anaesthesia, it is usual to see colours and vague shapes and to hear the noise of the equipment and operating staff during the operation. One member of the staff is designated to care for you and you can communicate with the staff if you are experiencing any problems.

After the operation

Your eye will be covered and you will be returned to the pre-operative area. It is usual to feel slight discomfort around the eye after cataract surgery but you must alert staff to severe pain. When you feel ready, the eye will be checked and you will be discharged home with contact telephone numbers, eye drops for the following week, an eye clinic review appointment, and a letter for your doctor.

Leave the eye dressing alone until the following morning, when it may be removed. It is common to notice better sight immediately, although some have more gradual improvement over the following weeks. The "new" eye is vulnerable to being banged and care must be taken to protect it. Otherwise, it can be used immediately for reading and watching television. Updated spectacles will be needed in time (4–6 weeks after operation) for more accurate focus. If the vision is good enough, driving is permitted as soon as full recovery from the anaesthesia has occurred. There are no contraindications to flying and you may return to desk-work within a week.

Appendix C: Checklist for surgical decisions

Criterion	YES – Options	NO – Options
Does the patient agree to have regional anaesthesia?	List for regional anaesthesia	Book appointment for general anaesthetic pre-assessment clinic
Does the patient understand English?	List for regional anaesthesia	Either arrange interpreter for day of surgery, or consider general anaesthesia
Does patient have companion at home?	Ambulatory care (AC)	AC – if patient is fit to be alone on first postoperative night (with telephone), or if a temporary companion can be found for night of surgery, or low dependency overnight stay.
Does patient have independent transport?	Ambulatory care (AC)	AC – if transport can be arranged or low dependency overnight stay

Appendix D: Discharge scoring system

Vital signs
2 = within 20% of preoperative value
1 = within 20–40% of preoperative value
0 = within 40% of preoperative value

Activity and mental status
2 = orientated in time, place and person **and** steady gait
1 = orientated in time, place and person **or** steady gait
0 = neither

Pain, nausea and/or vomiting
2 = minimal
1 = moderate
0 = severe

Surgical bleeding
2 = none
1 = minimal
0 = moderate

Intake and output
2 = taking oral fluids, has urinated
1 = **either** taking oral fluids, **or** has urinated
0 = neither

Score >8 = fit for discharge
<8 = unfit for discharge (refer on)

Appendix E: Typical discharge advice to patients after day case cataract surgery

- We suggest that you spend a quiet evening at home following your cataract surgery.
- Your eye will feel a little bruised this evening, and we recommend that you take simple painkillers to relieve any discomfort you may feel as the anaesthetic wears off.
- You may eat and drink normally, although if you have had a general anaesthetic today, we recommend a light supper and you should avoid alcohol.
- Take care not to bang your eye.
- Your eye shield and dressing should remain in place until tomorrow morning.
- Your next clinic appointment is .... (day), at .... (time), at .... (site).
- If you have severe eye pain, or pain that is not relieved by simple painkillers, this may indicate that there is a problem with your eye. In the first instance, please try to contact the eye team.
- During normal working hours phone the eye clinic on ....(eye clinic, nurse station). Alternatively please phone ....(hospital switchboard) and ask for the eye doctor on call.
- If the pain is persistent we shall need to see you to check that the eye is safe.
- Out-of-hours we will need you to come to the casualty department, ...(address) which is open 24 hours a day.
- Please bring this letter and the day-unit discharge letter with you and show them to the receptionist at the front desk.
- If you need to contact your GP tonight, please show them the discharge letter so that they will know about your eye surgery.

Index